Keeping our Children Healthy

Holistic care

for future generations

Angela Bea

Previous books by Angela Bea

Self-help Fibromyalgia - your body will heal itself

A concise self-help book for those wishing to overcome the pain of Fibromyalgia

Right Thinking, Right Doing

An overview from birth to death on Healthy Living for us and the planet

Natural pregnancy and Childcare

A journey from conception to school age, with many helpful tried and tested tips from a midwife and mother. This next book creates a natural sequel to this one.

All available on Amazon.co.uk and Kindle

This book is dedicated to all those children, including my own three very special ones, who have taught me so much on my life journey as a parent, nanny and carer.

Contents

Disclaimer:

All the information and advice given in this book is not an alternative to seeking medical advice when necessary. Any diet, treatment or advice in this book is given purely as another mother's opinion and is not to be taken as 'professional advice.' It is the parent's ultimate responsibility where they seek and find help for their children.

Angela Bea 2013

Introduction

During the writing of my last book 'Natural Pregnancy and Childcare, holistic insights of a mother and midwife' many of my life experiences as a midwife, maternity nurse and nanny kept coming up in my memories. I also began dipping more and more into the deep well of **instinctual knowledge** which I have been practicing all my working life and which is there for everyone to access.

This knowledge is often hidden from sight nowadays. Maternal Instincts are getting forgotten, as we discover more and more scientific phenomena and rely more and more on the 'demigods' which we have created in the guise our GP's, health visitors, practice nurses and Paediatricians, who tell us how to bring up our children and keep them safe and healthy.

Added to these professionals, who sincerely believe they are doing a good job, I would also like to add the hidden and sometimes sinister influence of the drug companies and the financial pressures which are put on governments and health departments by these to sell products to keep us 'healthy'.

We are being brainwashed more and more to believe, through the media, many parenting magazines, advertising and general 'knowledge' (wherever that stems from), that without dosing up our children when they get minor illnesses, disinfecting everything from 'germs', and living in a certain way as modern parents, then our children will be put at risk and we will have another pandemic 'plague' or even death on our hands!

This may sound a bit extreme, but look into the average family's First Aid and home medicine kit and you will be shocked at the number of pills and potions which have found their way there at some crisis moment, and which are probably out of date and waiting to poison your children next time they feel unwell.

The aim of this book is to give parents, grannies, nannies and others involved with children's care the oportunity to look at **common sense, tried and tested** means of **staying healthy**, rather than treating when the children get ill.

It also includes some Granny's Remedies and self-help treatments, which may have been forgotten by your family.

As a retired nurse I know that illness and disability in our children is a stark reality and there are times when modern science does its work in saving lives. I have worked in hospital wards with critically ill children. This book honours what is done to help in these situations.

However there are many, many times when a child is taken along to the GP unnecessarily because the parent **does not have the confidence** or knowhow to see what is truly happening to their offspring and give support and love in that process.

My hope is to give a useful reference guide and a thought provoking read to those parents who would like to relink to their instinctual knowledge and learn to care for their children in a more natural way.

Illness need not be frightening. It is OUR OWN fear which colours the situation, and by remaining fearless we give protection to the child going through a process.

In each of my books thus far I refer to **Universal Energy**. It is the Essence of Life, Movement and Growth and is an integral part of everything. If we can become conscious of how we access it, loose it, share it and depend on it for Health, we can start to understand how many modern day practices are in fact **depriving** human beings of this Energy and we become like hot-house plants which have not had enough light and air and nourishment.

Energy is not just sunshine, although it is related to this; it is not just LOVE, but we can ponder on this word in the broadest sense; it is LIFE which in its Religious context may be referred to as GOD, or GOOD. Keeping it simple, I prefer to call it Universal Energy. Some cultures call it CHI, others PRANA. It is neither 'religious' nor 'spiritual', but is just a common fact of our existence which has not been named or recognised by science (as it is taught in schools at present); however most modern cutting edge scientists are very close to understanding it.

It has many different levels of 'integration' with our physical body; it joins with our most dense physical structure or matter, where it can be found in the interchange of substances at cellular level; it creates movement and energy when we run round; it enables us to experience human emotions, and the deep Love felt by a parent for its child, and gives the growing child a sense of its own Self.

It enables us to change, grow, develop and reach our greatest potential as human beings. The absence of it can be acutely felt in a deprived child, unloved and unnurtured.

This Energy is what I shall be making you aware of throughout this book.

As this is strictly speaking a sequel to the last book on **Natural Pregnancy and Childcare**, may I suggest that you read that one first, to avoid unnecessary repetition of the basics, which I will refer to again and again.

Why a problem

'**Illness**' is a nasty word and has certain connotations of pain, hospitals, being out of control, visits to the doctor, taking nasty tasting medicines, and life generally stopping while we sit tight to make sure we don't die!

'**Health**' has other connotations, the main things being; feeling pain free, full of **Energy,** able to run around and perform everything we want to, able to eat and drink whatever we want, feeling positive that we will go on for ever like this.

'**Healing**' is the hope that we are getting back to a place of health.

Our life experiences colour how we feel about these three words. We may ourselves have had a nasty bout of illness as a young child and the dreamlike memories of fear, pain and concerned adults, with maybe even a separation from our parents, give us a sense of foreboding or fear.

Just for a moment stop and remember your own 'childhood illnesses' or accidents, which you felt were major events on your journey through childhood.

Do you remember being afraid? Where you perhaps rushed off to a strange frightening hospital? Or was it pleasant to stay at home off school with your Mum, Dad or Granny taking care of you and bringing you perhaps bowls of jelly, thinly sliced bread and butter, or a special piece of fruit. Were you allowed to watch a special TV programme or snuggle up in your parent's bed, or look at a treasured book to while away the long hours? Do you remember being delirious from a fever, or taking nasty tasting medicines?

These experiences and memories will strongly affect how you deal with your own children's illnesses and health problems. If I am opening up some skeletons in the cupboard it is for the very reason that our FEAR will influence how we can deal with and help to heal our children.

Young babies come into this world with no expectations of life except those that have been inherited via the genetic makeup and those felt in utero during pregnancy from the mother. I make a strong case that any major trauma occurring during pregnancy WILL have a subconscious effect on the unborn child at some level. Therefore, again, remember what happened during the child's development in utero. Were you as a pregnant mother happy and fulfilled, or anxious and unwell with lots of major life upheavals? This will have a bearing on your child's ability to cope with any events in the future, and whether they associate 'stresses' with fear.

I would like to bring this pondering one stage further and take a stance which you may like to encompass or reject outright as ridiculous! That is, that we come to earth many times and our previous memories are held deep within us at an Energetic level.

Reincarnation, as this is known, has been accepted by many people all over the planet for many thousands of years. There are modern anecdotal instances of children remembering a past life and traumas and if this is so, it may also colour the relationship they have to their body during this incarnation, and what they experience in this life as 'lessons' on a soul level. I leave you with this thought!

Another aspect you may become interested in is the idea that all Energy in the Universe is interconnected, and therefore at conception, and also at the baby's first breath, this pattern of Energy *imprints* itself on the child as an influence of Cosmic Energy. This is known as a birth chart and is unique to each individual. Patterns of the planets and fixed stars have been studied for many thousands of years and are known as Astrology. If looked at and read in an intuitive broad way they can shed light on many difficulties, gifts and qualities which make up the child's destiny and character.

So here you have the full picture of the influences on your child's development;

- Chance!
- Genetic inheritance
- 'Nature or nurture'
- The mind/body connection
- Karma, or the influence of our deeds in a previous lifetime
- Astrological influences

You can decide which of these aspects is meaningful in your path together with your growing child. This will also colour how you think about illness if it occurs.

The 'meaning of illness' is an area which is now being explored more and more by general medicine, as the mind/body connection becomes more accepted.

Thus 'We create what we are and have, in terms of life patterns and illnesses'. So **illness is** nothing more than **an expression and reaction of the body to what has been happening around it in the previous weeks, months or years.**

This latter viewpoint is what I will base this book on, as it is easily acceptable to everyman and does not pose heavy philosophical questions.

However as a parent, experience brings untold wisdom and when something happens that you cannot understand you may be led to ponder it more deeply in order to understand its meaning.

The body has the innate ability to come to a point of BALANCE and does this by **creating a state of illness** which then gives the organism **time** and **energy** to come back to that central point of balance. Illness is the **means** by which we become whole again! It can therefore be seen as a helpful blessing rather than an ill-fated wind.

For each individual this central point of balance will be a different place, which means there is no 'correct way' of dealing with, for example, the common cold, as a tall thin sensitive person will deal with it differently from a short fat fiery person. We are all 'constitutionally' unique and therefore there is no ideal human being, or 'perfect health'. What works for one will be wrong for another.

In Chinese medicine, Ayurveda medicine and other Holistic approaches, such as Homeopathy and Anthroposophic medicine, the WHOLE PERSON is carefully observed before any treatment is given.

How this 'Balancing of the Life Energies' is going to be supported by natural remedies is the science of these aforementioned approaches, and as such can be respected, once one understands that the whole human being is being treated not just the symptoms, as is the case in allopathic medicines which you get from the GP or the chemist.

Therefore searching out these alternative treatments for your children not only ensures that they do not have to suffer the poisoning side effects of drugs given to them, but their bodily processes are supported naturally when their own bodies are trying to heal themselves, coming back to that unique point of balance, which for that individual at that particular time is **health.**

I wish you well on this path of exploration which is indeed a path of deep learning and is the gift our children can bring to us, their parents.

Conscious parenting is the most fulfilling and interesting path, and has huge consequences on the future of the planet as our offspring go out into life as strong healthy individuals. A healthy society creates a healthy future for our planet.

The World Health Organisation is the body that currently holds the responsibility and know-how for our future health. It looks at patterns of illness and future trends, based solely on what is happening now. By changing our attitudes and actions around the health of our children, we can change these assumptions built on statistics. We can prove that human beings have an amazing ability to adapt and change when circumstances force us to.

Never before have there been such huge changes taking place worldwide in human health; in attitudes and new possibilities for healing the planet.

As parents you can be at the forefront of these changes.

The Immune System

What do we understand by the Immune System? It is the most vital aspect of remaining healthy.

Over thousands of years our human bodies have built up a way of combatting foreign invasion of microbes, bacteria, viruses and fungal organisms which can be found around us in the environment and also within us. Put in simple terms we carry within us 'good' and 'bad' organisms, which often only become bad if they live in the wrong place in our bodies, or start to multiply massively creating an 'Illness'.

Within our circulating blood are cells which have developed specifically for fighting these invading inappropriate organisms, including white blood cells, specifically T cells, and others. They have the ability to engulf and swallow up malignant organisms, and it is during this process of 'fighting infection', (or foreign cell activities such as cancer,) that the body reacts in a particular way.

Heat is engendered during this fight; an inflammatory process which we know as **FEVER.** During the course of a febrile illness, the temperature (which is normally between 36-37degrees centigrade) can rise as much as 3 or 4 degrees. The body also responds by using its lymphatic tissues, or glands, situated in the neck, armpits, abdomen and groin areas, to filter out the dead or infected cells and cleanse the body; a wonderful mechanism! The foreign organisms are literally 'burned out' by the body's heat.

In a simple febrile illness caused by a virus such as influenza there are other symptoms also, such as muscle achiness, headache, sore eyes, sore throat, perhaps sickness or diarrhoea. The whole body 'feels ill' and our first response nowadays is to suppress the fever with paracetamol or aspirin or some such drug, and try to stop the symptoms

The whole body is working hard to combat the infection and the only way to heal it fully is to **work with it.**

Rest, fluids, an alkaline diet (of which more later) and sleep will help the body to overcome its crisis and balance itself again. The usual course of a febrile illness is that the temperature drops again after a day or two, and even goes below normal for 24 hours, and the body will gradually rebalance itself and the symptoms will diminish, leaving the person weak but renewed and cleansed.

Time is the one factor which our modern society deprives the body of in this healing process. **The body needs time to heal.** If we rush it, by using antibiotics, anti-febrile drugs and pain killers we leave the body in a weakened state for the next invasion of bugs, rather like a defeated army being attacked again!

By allowing the body to heal itself, the body also becomes strengthened. It has produced **antibodies** to the particular bacteria, which will protect it if this invades again in the future. This is known as a Healthy Immune System, where the person builds up natural immunity to common illnesses and the bacteria which can often be found, particularly in wintertime, in damp or muggy crowded spaces.

Common colds are perhaps the exception to this, as we can catch them frequently, but if we are healthy and unstressed we do not catch colds, even if people sneeze in our faces. We manage to overcome the ingested virus before it gives us symptoms with our immune system.

Mothers pass their accrued antibodies on to their children, in utero, and more particularly in the first breast milk, known as Colostrum. It is very important that babies get this milk as otherwise they are much more likely to contract the common illnesses in their society, such as flu, coughs and tummy bugs, and also any of the 'childhood illnesses' which their mother has had herself.

Genetic inheritance is an important aspect of illness and when a homeopath or doctor takes a full history, they always ask in detail about the parents' and grandparents' illnesses, particularly things like cancer and TB.

As children grow and become more mobile they will naturally contact bacteria in the environment, as in dirt and soil, and will start to build immunity against these. A healthy child will be naturally immune to many illnesses by the time it starts to mix with many other children at about aged 3.

But something is not right here, I hear you say! We are told to cleanse and disinfect things to stop infection. Keeping everything squeaky clean has been found in recent studies to increase our chances of catching common illnesses, as natural immunity does not get the right stimulation to develop.

Nowadays we are being told to have our children immunised against many sometimes fatal illnesses. Otherwise they may die of horrible complications or get brain damage, or go blind or deaf.

The government's immunisation programme starts ever earlier and small babies are now receiving multiple injections to stop them from getting these diseases: these listed below are the most common, but this list is not finite, neither are the side effects which may occur.

Illness	Vaccination	Possible side effect
• Measles, mumps, rubella,	(MMR)	Eczema, autism
• Diphtheria, tetanus, pertussis	(DTP)	
• Haemophilus influenza	(HIB)	Diabetes
• Hepatitis B	(HBV)	Multiple sclerosis
• Pneumococcus	(PVC)	
• Meningitis	(MCV4)	
• Varicella		
• Polio		

The 'American Academy of Paediatrics' has an interesting website which shows just how far this Immunisation programme has progressed and all the injections currently available, and being given to most children.

In England there are strong financial incentives from the government for GPs to get a 100% take-up for childhood vaccinations.

But what about the claims that there are side effects?

It is claimed that since the '80's, when the government programmes were fully established, the numbers of antigens in vaccines has been reduced considerably, making them ever safer.

The arguments about the causes of infantile autism go on! It is now thought that the mercury used in producing the vaccines may be the main cause of autism.

As a discerning parent how does one start to take the very important decision as to whether to have your child immunised against all these diseases, or to refuse this service or to make a compromise with just a few of them, and if so which ones?

It is one of the first major decisions that one makes for the child after birth, (other than whether to breast or bottle feed), and has far reaching consequences on the health and life of the child right up into adulthood.

Finding out as much as possible about the different illnesses and how prevalent they still are in your area is an important starting point. One could argue that this is a selfish standpoint, not to vaccinate, as the disease only becomes 'extinct' if you do 100% vaccination programmes. The aim of vaccination programmes is to obliterate these diseases!

But a strange phenomenon can be observed here. New diseases come along in the place of the old ones! It is as though the bacteria or virus develops its own immune system and fights back to survive.

The same is the case with the use of antibiotics, which since the last world war have become used more and more to fight the multiplying of bacteria in the body. There are now more and more 'superbugs' to be found in hospital environments, and some professionals are warning that antibiotics may become useless in the future as a new generation of bugs are born. Bugs have learnt to survive too!

I believe that if too many immunizations are given and too many antibiotics used, the Energy of the child and their Immune System becomes severely compromised and this can give rise to illnesses in later life, such as ME, Chronic fatigue and Fibromyalgia as well as an increase in allergies.

Having suffered from the latter myself I can trace the onset of it to a large dose of travel immunisations I had in mid-life which, combined with stress, so compromised my immune system that it went into a virtual shutdown. It took many years of careful diet and lifestyle changes to come back to a state of health and it is still vulnerable to stress.

Interestingly vets recognise a condition known as 'Vacinosis' in animals, but it has yet to be recognised by the medical profession. I suspect there is too much financial payoff at stake for them to take this seriously at present.

With my own three children, my husband and I decided only to give them Tetanus vaccine, which is active in Gloucestershire in the ground. We had an allotment and the children spent a lot of time playing out in the garden and fields. It was MY FEAR which made me go that route. I only started the course once they were fully mobile and playing outside, at about aged 3.They had all the childhood illnesses, (whooping cough, measles, rubella, mumps, and chicken pox) and I nursed them through them. My daughter prides herself at never having taken a single allopathic drug and she is now 32!

All three of them travelled widely as they became adults and we discussed which jabs were essential for each country they were visiting, and they had only those absolutely necessary. Some of my friends and colleagues think I did a disservice to the general immunity of the population by not giving them their jabs. The debate continues!

Acidity and alkalinity

I would now like to mention specifically the work of **Dr Robert Young**, an American biochemist whom I have met. He has researched over many years the life of blood, cells, bacteria, viruses, fungi, cancer cells and microbes in the blood under different environments of **acidity and alkalinity.** His popular book**, The pH Miracle,** describes what happens in the blood when we eat particular foods and act in certain ways to create over-acidity, which in turn encourages the over multiplication of 'malignant' cells of different kinds. If you put those same cells back into an **alkaline** environment they **revert back to healthy cells**, and the symptoms of illness disappear. There is a lot of further information about this approach to health on the website www.energiseforhealth.com which is an English version of the American www.innerlight.com including the work of Dr Young.

These research facts become an important key to understanding illness, and acting upon this knowledge can help keep us healthy. If we can stay alkaline we have a much higher chance of combatting infections, cancers and other chronic conditions such as Candida, Diabetes, Arthritis and Fibromyalgia.

Having virtually cured myself of Fibromyalgia over several years, I can vouch that if I become acidic because of stress, anger, eating the wrong foods or tiredness, then my body becomes acidic (as proved by urine pH tests) and my symptoms reappear. I am also much more likely to catch a cold. I have been doing research over several years on this, using my own body!

We can discover **what we can do ourselves** to improve our immune system, keep fit and well and avoid the many common viral infections which seem to attack those with a weak immune system, particularly if one is stressed or unhappy or it is cold and damp.

Returning to the gritty problem of whether or not to follow a full immunization programme with your children, try to understand the immune system in terms of Energy. A healthy supply of Energy from the Universe in the form of good food, right exercise, right thinking and a healthy emotional environment, enough sleep, avoiding many common toxins in today's environment, will give your child a strong start in combatting infections and will vastly reduce their **NEED for immunisation**.

Only you as a parent know whether you are **strong enough** to give your child these health-giving Energising elements in their day-to-day life, and whether you can overcome your **FEAR** of disease sufficiently to protect your child in other ways. Do not underestimate the role of fear in any disease! Fear stimulates the adrenals to produce cortisones and this in turn creates more acid in your blood.

The blood itself is extremely good at maintaining 'homeostasis', (or an even acid/alkaline environment,) but it does this at the cost of the body's organs, cells, joints etc., which can then become overly acidic and create illnesses. Therefore acidity does not show up in blood tests, unless one is seriously ill.

Ask any parent and they will naturally want to do 'the best' for their child, but much ignorance exists today as to what a healthy lifestyle consists of, which will enable children to develop healthy immune systems and fight off diseases themselves.

By taking full responsibility for your child's health and refusing immunisation programmes, you will also have to take the responsibility for providing an excellent diet, a relaxed happy lifestyle with plenty of fresh air, exercise and love to give the child the best start in life and build a healthy immune system.

Nature or nurture?

This question has become something of a cliché in our society, but it begs the question how as parents do you give your children the 'best environment'?

If children are asthmatic or have eczema, for example, this may be from a long line of **genetic inheritance** and it may be a 'family weakness' which is already known about before conception In this case it will be doubly important to address it consciously during pregnancy or even before you get pregnant, and decide whether you will adopt special exclusion diet during pregnancy, cut out all alcohol, wheat, diary, caffeine, sugar and artificial additives, if you do not know what the specific allergens are. If there is a family history of nut allergy, for example, you can omit these. The process which produces allergens is complex but often starts in utero.

Being **aware of inherited family illnesses, from both sides of the family** is therefore important in preconception and pregnancy care. It may be wise to see if the treatments you are getting for an 'Illness' yourself can be modified during pregnancy so that you do not have active symptoms. Try to cut out all medications if you can and go to a holistic practitioner for help and advice. This might be a Naturopath, Homeopath, Acupuncturist or Ayurveda practitioner.

You may have a stomach weakness of some kind for example, IBS or a tendency to ulcers. This could also be inherited, so it is important to look again at what upsets your stomach and change your diet accordingly.

Nervous conditions are very common, and anxieties around childbirth may highlight something that happened at your own birth, so addressing that with the help of hypnosis or counselling may be a good idea.

If you are unfortunate enough to have suffered from a cancerous illness this could also be due to your lifestyle or environment in some way. Are you living near an environmentally polluting nuclear power station or overhead power lines, or near a motorway or other disturbance? Is it possible to remedy this in some way before the pregnancy is too far advanced, by moving house?

Look carefully at your own lifestyle and diet. Are you smoking, which has been proven to cause bronchitis and asthma in infants? Do you use a microwave and eat only frozen ready meals, which have little Energy in them? How much organic food can you source and eat?

I have covered many of these aspects in my book 'Natural pregnancy and childcare,' so if you have health problems with your baby or child, go back and read this and see what may have caused them. Remain alert to environmental, dietary and inherited problems as the child grows up. Have you missed a vital clue as to WHY they are creating these illness symptoms?

Stress is probably the greatest cause of illness in our modern children. It comes in many forms but is a sad fact of our modern lives. We travel around in cars, planes and trains, we sit for hours in front of moving images on the TV, Nintendo or screen games and computer, we have many financial stresses which may well be 'absorbed' unconsciously by our children.

Relationship problems often go along with all these things, to the extent that 2/3 of children nowadays may have to cope with a divorce situation, step parents, or half-siblings, and two homes. Often one or other parent may be absent completely and many many children are partially brought up by nannies or child-minders or in nurseries because our society and government is currently encouraging all mothers to go out to work. This may be a financial necessity for some, but society's 'norms' are very hard to go against.

All these things have a bearing on our children's health. In the 'bad old days' there was lack of health-care, schooling, lack of sanitation, cold damp houses, extreme poverty and hunger, even the dreaded workhouse.

Fortunately many of these things have improved (although the current financial situation in Britain means that many families are again going into poverty). If a child does not have enough good food, light and exercise and most importantly a sense of security and being loved, then they will start to show signs of illness.

These signs of stress may appear first in small ways like poor sleep quality, poor appetite, bedwetting and then go on to show more serious things such as restlessness, bad behaviour, disruption at school, increased coughs, colds and tummy upsets, abnormal fevers, glue ear or headaches. The child may even become depressed or suicidal or may go on to develop some major symptoms such as severe asthma, epilepsy, childhood arthritis, diabetes or cancer.

Major illness does not just happen! It is the **final outcome** of a situation which may have been developing over several years and as such can be traced backwards by a discerning parent or practitioner. When and how and most importantly WHY did these symptoms start? Why has the child been stressed, or was it neglectful diet or lifestyle which pushed the child into illness?

As parents caring for children we need to stay alert at all times as to how we have been acting with and treating our children. Many illnesses can be avoided by simple changes in diet and lifestyle, and if you are not coping with life and things are getting too stressful this can have a direct impact on the health of your children. It may seem obvious that a happy secure environment is also a healthy environment, but what changes can YOU make now to improve it yet further and ensure that your children stay as healthy as possible not just as children but into adulthood, because as parents this is our ultimate responsibility; to ensure a healthy and happy future generation.

Whatever inherited problems are encountered it is still possible to help the child to heal and grow strong through healthy nurture.

Another simpler interpretation of Nature and Nurture can be based around our most **basic human needs.**

These can be listed as;

- Good nourishment
- Light and fresh air
- Protection from adverse climatic conditions and enemies
- Enablement and love

I will take each of these elements for survival and thriving and elaborate on them. We take much of this for granted but it is helpful to go back to these basics from time to time to see where we might be going very wrong in modern society.

Good Nourishment

Taking the idea of there being Universal Energy in ourselves and all around in Nature a step further, one can understand how taking in food is in fact taking in Energy from plants and animals and *transforming it for our own needs.* This, which we usually call digestion, is a magic process, far more complex than just the digestive enzymes which we learn about at school. The gut has a huge surface area and also 'intelligence' and if it becomes sick or inflamed it is the first thing which causes illness in us. It KNOWS what the body needs and can sort out the fine substances from the rubbish which we eat, and absorb just what the body needs at any particular time.

How stressed our intestines must be at present with all the rubbish that we try to put down there; chemical additives, large amounts of gluten, sugars, poisons off the land, even pollutants such as chlorine and fluoride which are added to our drinking water! Our poor gut is working extremely hard but in many instances becomes inflamed and the tiny Villae are damaged by too much of the wrong foodstuffs, even from an early age. If the gut is unhealthy then illnesses will follow.

Thus in fact we may be living with malnourishment when we think and hope we are eating 'healthily,' but not taking enough care of <u>what</u> we eat. We do not then have the capacity to absorb the right amounts of minerals, vitamins, proteins, good fats, carbohydrates and pure water into our systems and we suffer from food intolerances, obesity and other serious illnesses as we get older.

In the western world this has now reached epidemic proportions. In other parts of the world, where there is severe lack of food, the digestion has not got enough good food to imbibe and therefore also suffers. Parasites may also be a huge problem. In my book 'Right Thinking, Right Doing' I go into details about how to stay healthy by only eating the best quality and type of foods which the body craves.

If you want your children to grow up into healthy active adults then nourishment is the core factor of bringing them up. Spend time researching this subject even before you decide to have children, and resist copying the 'norm' of how we feed our children in the western world.

School meals have recently been in the press. Huge improvements are still needed here. It is much safer to provide your child with a healthy lunchbox which you can oversee.

A simple totally organic diet, taking **the plant as the basis for each meal**, is a good starting point for providing a healthy balanced meal. Each part of the plant has a different way of producing Energy.

1. **Roots** (carrots, beetroot, and parsnips for example) have stored Energy over the winter, and are therefore high in sugars and carbohydrates for energy.
2. **The stem** and leaves of plants give a balance of vitamins and minerals and are essential to health. They also absorb much light when growing, and therefore much Energy (e.g. cabbage, celery, salads)
3. **The flower** comes at the peak of the Energetic life of the plant, and usually in the time of greatest warmth. Its Energy is therefore huge. Plants such as broccoli and cauliflower are therefore most nutritious.
4. **The seed or fruit** is the Energy held ready for the next generation and as such also contain sugars and proteins. They are readily available as apples, grapes, citrus fruits, berries and so on (containing large amounts of instant Energy as Fructose) and **nuts and seeds**, which contain a lot of protein too. **Grains** also come into this category, and are used widely for their sustaining Energy (carbohydrate).

If one can create a balanced meal containing all of these 4 elements as shown above, from the plant world, then one has a good start in life and a much better chance to remain healthy.

A healthy lunchbox might therefore include some carrot sticks, celery, lettuce or watercress, raw broccoli, nuts or seeds or wholemeal bread with seed spread and a fruit! How often do you see a child eating this? If you start right, when children are first experiencing new tastes, it is easier to go on in this way. (Refer to Natural Pregnancy and Childcare for weaning and dietary tips)

Meat and fish, eggs and cheese and other dairy foods can be added in moderation to bring variety, but **they are not as essential as the right vegetable/fruit mix.**

If meat is eaten then it should be of a good quality and organic, locally reared and humanely slaughtered, as the meat industry is currently very suspect in adding hormones and antibiotics to animal feeds. Most animals are slaughtered in a fearful environment after long journeys, and the meat contains many stress hormones from that. Added to this problem are the other things like preservatives, and antioxidants, not to mention the ubiquitous horse meat!

Fish may be sourced from unknown highly polluted waters, and may contain heavy metals. Small fish, caught locally, are best. Try to buy fish that is sustainably caught. Fish contains good Omega oils, but these can be taken from seeds as well.

Dairy foods, including cheese, unless organically prepared, are nearly all full of growth hormones and may contain other additives, and they may also create a lot of mucous, so are best **avoided if your child has a blocked or runny nose, asthma, coughs or ear problems.** Alternatives to milk are coconut, almond, soya (but no GMO), rice, oat or goat's products, all organically grown. Always read the labels for hidden ingredients.

We still assume that milk is the most important food for young children. That *is* the case with breast milk of course, but why do we assume cows are able to provide best nourishment for our children? Their milk is created for their calves!

Eggs can be eaten sometimes but chose those organically grown; again the feedstuffs for chicken normally contain loads of artificial chemicals, antibiotics and hormones.

Grains, which make up a large proportion of our diet in the western world, should only be eaten in their original wholegrain form, as refined flour which is found in pastas, biscuits, white and dyed brown bread, cakes and pancakes has little nutritional value and can even cause obesity and diabetes. The **GI diet** which is based on how quickly foods are digested is a good one for daily living and will ensure you get enough of the right nutrients and reduce the fat-forming foods.

Oils are necessary for building up cell walls but they should be good quality olive oils, or other plant oils such as hemp or almond. Oils also can be found in fish. Omegas, found in oils, are essential for brain power. Consider giving your child omega supplements, but ensure they contain 3, 6, and 9 in the right balance.

Food of organic/biodynamic quality may be hard to come by and more expensive, but it is the best start in life you can give your dear ones. Several companies are now available online providing healthy locally grown organic food, and this can be delivered as a weekly box or separate order. Try to buy as locally as you can to avoid food miles.

Sugar is a poison to the body, but amazingly in added to most processed foods and we are therefore unwittingly eating huge quantities of it, unless you stop to read the labels, and only cook with basic fresh ingredients.

All this advice may sound extreme but only by demanding unadulterated food will things start to change for the better and our children will not have such obesity problems and be overall healthier. YOU can vote with your feet and put pressure on governments and farmers to begin to grow healthier food for us all. This will, in the longer term, also benefit the planet's health, as the soil will become richer, and food will again contain the vitamins and minerals it used to. Currently many supermarket vegetables have little nutritional value! It is not just about large crops and cheaper prices!

Thinking about other aspects of agriculture, one can also muse on the difference in the health of cows kept in overcrowded conditions on factory farms, producing large quantities of milk, or the health of cows on mixed farms, where animals, grains and vegetables are all grown together in a balanced way.

A good example of this type of organic farm is Highgrove, in Gloucestershire, belonging to Prince Charles, where the land is sustained with organic muck and the crops are balanced, without the use of chemicals. It is the very hard labour-intensive methods which produce the best results, and we seem to have lost the ability to honour hard work in this country. Our children are being educated to sit in offices in front of computers! Rates of pay reflect our society's priorities.

Having your own garden and growing your own vegetables is not only satisfying and fun, but also produces the best food! It is grown with love and your Energy. You and your family are relating to a local patch of the earth and are caring and sustaining nature throughout the seasons. This is healing in itself both to the planet and us. The allotments in cities have become more and more popular in recent years, which is a sign of hope for the future.

This is nourishment for our children which we can become proud of! Fresh is best.

"Pick 'em and eat 'em", straight off the plant if possible! Learn to forage for wild plants too. There is plenty out in nature fit to eat. Make sure you are well informed about what you are finding out in nature, especially with fungi. There are some excellent books available now on foraging.

Light and fresh air

Strangely this is an issue which is much less spoken about, but equally as important as nutrition in maintaining good health generally.

When we go outside on a sunny day and run around we are soaking up the oxygen and sunlight into our bodies and this will act as an Energetic 'sponge' for growth and Energy. Notice how quickly your hair and finger nails grow in a warmer climate.

Interestingly there are some people on this planet who have become so spiritually developed that they no longer have to eat food, but can **survive on Light alone**! This proves the phenomenon that we do absorb Energy from the sun, and can even live off this, taking in no food whatsoever. It is not to be tried out without proper preparation and training however!

Strangely we have become so frightened of the sun that our children are in serious danger of not getting enough of it. We are scared of skin cancer and we wrap our children up in plastic when they go out in summer, putting on thick sun block creams and plastic playsuits on the beach to 'protect them'. I am NOT saying that children should be allowed to burn, far from it, but a little and often is the best way.

When we have sunny days in early spring or autumn it is so important to get out for a play or walk, and not sit around indoors or in school. A daily walk in all seasons to and from school is healthy and good. How many of our children now are taken by car everywhere and rarely go into the countryside to play, or run around in the garden, even in winter?

Exercise encourages good blood and lymph circulation and exchange of oxygen in the cells. It helps excretion of waste products too and maintains our weight and muscular strength. It enables bones to stay strong and not become brittle and is health-giving in every sense of the word. It relaxes the mind and enables us to de-stress, concentrate and learn better too.

Daily exercise is a vital part of remaining healthy. Muscles start to deteriorate after only 6 hours of not being used.

Children are naturally boisterous and enjoy running around and moving as soon as they are able to take an active part in the world. Firstly as babies they learn to wave their limbs around, especially when naked, to roll over, and sit up, then they come up onto their knees and pull themselves up onto furniture or an adults hand, and then one day, having walked with help for some weeks, they suddenly 'take off' independently and become toddlers.

All baby animals have this natural instinct. Watch a young lamb, goat or calf, just after it has been born, and see the effort it takes to totter along on trembling legs.

Within hours it is steady and soon will be jumping and gambolling amongst its friends out in the meadow. The Levitation and Energy of this movement is a joy to behold.

Watch young children in the park playing chase with each other, or running and jumping into puddles. It is natural for us to move in a healthy state.

Try staying absolutely still for some time and you will begin to feel how the cells and blood are still moving within the body. Movement is LIFE. Life is MOVEMENT.

As parents we can encourage this movement in a healthy and harmonious way. Non-jerky non-aggressive dance is wonderful to do and watch. Why do modern dancers do this popular jerky movement? Is it because we are losing touch with this natural harmony of movement and we need heavy beat rhythm to stimulate us to move at all?

The Olympic tradition of the Games can indeed be encouraged amongst young people as running, jumping, throwing, swimming, riding, jousting and other sports are all natural easy movements which if practised in a non-forceful way can bring us into a healthy relationship with our bodies. In health we are at ease with our bodies. We enjoy the movement. Team games can also encourage this.

So as soon as you become parents think about what exercise you do yourselves, and how to incorporate a healthy life-style into life as a family. Can you take a country walk at the weekend; ensure you have holidays with plenty of sunshine and running around, with not too many hours in the car? Can you take the children out every day to a park or countryside area, without car fumes, noise and danger? Much better to incorporate something natural than rush the kids off to the mini-gym after school in the car.

Many people nowadays live in cities, but planners know our physical needs for exercise, space and green parks and they are always to be found somewhere. Even walking around an estate can be a time for observing the changes in the gardens. Walking in nature can become a fun family time.

When our children were little we used to go out at least twice a week for a good long walk in the woods, or hills and now they are adult they still practice this.

Protection from adverse climatic conditions and enemies

This may sound an obvious thing in our society nowadays, but it is the most basic form of security for a growing child; to have a home which it knows and loves, which can become its own creative space and haven.

In our current society in Britain many children are living in temporary accommodation, bed and breakfast establishments, or with grandparents, as there is a real housing crisis, caused by over-inflation of house prices, high rentals and lack of council houses. This has become a political nightmare for many, and now the Government is planning to build over many acres of England's 'Green and pleasant land', destroying the very thing which keeps us healthy! What a short-sighted crazy idea!

At the same time there are thousands of empty properties around the country, under-occupied houses, (as many people now live on their own) and many 2nd homes which stand empty for much of the year.

Greedy landlords are allowed to push up rentals much higher than mortgages for equivalent properties, and mortgages are very hard to come by, as a self-employed person, or first time buyer. We urgently need new legislation on these issues.

This state of affairs has meant a lot of stress for poorer families, which has had a direct effect on children's health.

'Enemies' can also be interpreted as danger and criminal offences on our streets, caused by social deprivation, very mixed races and classes within communities, who rely heavily on the welfare state for survival and high unemployment in these areas. Things seem to be getting worse at present with government policies.

A way forward can only be found when communities themselves start to take responsibility for their own members and act together as a whole to upgrade empty houses, grow food on community allotments and city farms, become more neighbourly and loving, and act strongly in order to discipline destructive youths, who are bored, frustrated and angry with this degrading society.

In other countries 'enemies' are real life-threatening terrorists, or worse still government soldiers, who are heavily armed by us in the west. The only way forward towards peaceful solutions and health for our children worldwide is by banning firearms and ammunitions, in fact ceasing to produce them at all, and helping communities to rebuild their lives from total destruction. This may take several generations of loving care and guidance to achieve. Wars could cease, if we all believed strongly enough in non-violence. Idealistic? No, true!

'Adverse climatic conditions' are affecting most countries of the world in some form nowadays, as we seem to get more extreme weather patterns, with no immediate solutions. Until we learn to balance our own lives and live in a more ecological way day to day, reducing the use of cars, using less fossil fuels, and polluting less, our planet will continue to be 'sick'. Our children are the next generation and can be taught about the problems which we have created for them and some possible solutions which are emerging from are cutting edge scientists, designers and ecologists.

Schools take an active role here, but enlightened parents can also guide their children towards a better, healthier future.

Enabling and LOVE

This last thing on my list encompasses the real meaning of parenting. What do I mean by Enabling? It is allowing the incarnating child to develop into a strong and confident human being with unique gifts and qualities, which may appear 'out of the blue' or seem to be inherited from a parent or grandparent. Children, if given love and guidance in the right measure, whilst also being given firm boundaries, will develop into individuals with minds and souls of their own, to go out into life and develop into strong adults

How does one do this as a parent? Becoming ever less selfish, fearful and controlling, and more loving is the obvious path of development of a parent, but sometimes a hard School of Life. Nowadays there has been a swing towards more freedom and less discipline both at home and in the classroom. Is this necessarily the right way forward?

I sincerely believe that children with firm boundaries are more secure and will have fewer behaviour problems than those who are allowed to argue and get their own way when they have a tantrum, be that as a baby or teenager!. 'No' simply means 'no'! This starts in the cradle. How one treats a baby will then reflect in the toddler, in the preschool child, the school child and then the teenager. Start as you mean to go on!

Decide what rules are important in your household and practice them YOURSELVES and stick to them. This requires **self-discipline**, courage and humour, and most importantly a partnership in parenting. When parents have different attitudes in parenting and discipline, things can go awry.

Within a simple framework of rhythm and consistency the child can develop as an individual, be praised and encouraged in all they do creatively and lovingly, find their own means of expressing who they truly are and work through their own issues which become apparent as they mature. No human being is perfect and getting along with your children, warts and all, is as important as getting on with your partner!

This may all seem so obvious to you that it is hardly worth reading about, but you may come across a screaming child in a supermarket whose mother is about to abuse it verbally and physically, and a quiet encouraging word may help disperse the situation, or you may have a friend or relative going through a tough time with discipline or marital difficulties. We can all learn to help each other.

Keeping families healthy is a community affair. In African tribes if a couple is having a problem, a ritual is created where the whole village stands around the couple who are placed into a 'magic circle' and they listen and give advice and ask for the wisdom of the ancestors to come and help them.

In western society we can also perform this important task of listening and standing beside someone in a crisis. It is not necessarily about giving advice and trying to sort out the problem as just BEING there for them in a loving way.

The last word to be mentioned in terms of healthy living is LOVE.

"Love the Lord thy God and love Thy neighbour as Thyself" was Jesus' commandment to us. If we can understand this in its broadest context we have the 'recipe for a healthy family life', to enable our children to grow up and develop into happy healthy adults. This is a Christian Ethic, but can be applied to any creed or religious belief, or even Atheism!

It is NOT about beliefs and details of cultural traditions, but about **acceptance and love** of the rich variety which we have created as the human race. Here in Britain we are particularly diverse in race and cultures, so perhaps we, as the country from which I write, have a task to show the whole world how it is done?

Part 2

Practical aspects of Caring for a sick child at home

Common ailments

We have already looked at WHY a child may become ill, and avoidance of stress and overtiredness is of course the ideal. But children DO sometimes get poorly and need an environment and time for their bodies to rebalance and heal.

Keeping a child at home, where they have their own bed, familiar things around and the Energy of a loving mother and father is the very best thing you can do for a sick child.

Nowadays there is increasing pressure for women to go out to work and therefore this becomes the first problem when a child is 'under the weather'; who is to look after them?

Grandparents, if they live close enough, can perhaps act as a help in this scenario, and many young working mothers resort to this in a crisis. Nannies, who may already be employed, may act as 'surrogate' Mum in this situation and provide a calm and healing environment in the home.

The worst scenario is probably to send an unwell child off to nursery or school when really they should be kept quietly at home. 'Kalpol', children's Paracetamol, is often used in this situation to keep the child going, and suppress any fever which may develop. By doing this the child has to work even harder to heal and often the natural healing process is suppressed.

Chronic conditions then may develop, such as ear aches, chesty coughs which don't clear up, croup, tonsillitis, tummy aches, and headaches which keep recurring throughout the winter months, or towards the end of long school terms, when most children get more and more tired from long days spent indoors with little or no play/creative time.

The child is then taken to the doctor who prescribes antibiotics and the 'bug' is temporarily suppressed. The immune system however has been weakened by this treatment, and the illness may go to a deeper level and create allergies, chronic asthma/bronchitis, IBS, chronic fatigue, or even Rheumatoid arthritis, or cancer.

If a child is tired and stressed it will easily 'pick up a bug' from school or nursery. This bacterium or virus may already have been in the blood or tissues of the child for some time, but as the acidity of the child rises from stress the organism has the perfect environment to start growing and multiplying, causing symptoms.(refer back to acid and alkalinity in part 1.)

This may also happen to you as an adult when you 'keep going', seemingly healthily, but when you stop or go on holiday; then your body has the time to be ill, or rebalance itself. It happens commonly in people who push themselves too hard.

Any treatments given and home remedies for children should therefore always be aimed at **alkalising** the system. The following tips will hopefully give you, the parent, plenty of help without resorting to drugs.

The common cold and its complications

Colds can easily be 'caught' as our antibodies seem to forget how to protect us, even though we may have several colds in one year. They usually start with a sore throat, feeling tired and muzzy headed, and then the runny nose, sneezing, blocked sinuses and cough develop. At the beginning the best treatment is an early night, so the body can alkalise during sleep. The changes that occur in the cells during sleep ensure renewal and healing.

Lemon juice is an alkalising agent, strangely enough as it seems so acid, but a squeezed lemon in warm (not hot) water with a spoonful of good **local honey, which contains healing enzymes** stirred in and sipped slowly will ease a sore throat and reduce acidity.

Plenty of fluids are needed too, to help detoxify the body. Warm water is best, made into **herb tea** (peppermint, chamomile, sage are all good). Encourage children to take these drinks from babyhood and they will learn to accept them. Don't put sugar in as this is too acid. Rather use natural low GI sweetness, such as rice syrup or agave syrup if they do need a little sweetness.

All **fruits and vegetables** will help to alkalise the body, so try to offer as much of these as possible while the child is suffering from any kind of illness, in the form of vegetable soups, fruit puree (apple with berries is nice), or fresh fruit, cut into small pieces. Fresh stewed fruit is always better than the convenient sachets of fruit puree now widely available.

A super quick natural ice-cream can be made with chopped banana, put into a container in the freezer to harden. Berries and other fruits (mango and pear work well) can be frozen too to add colour and flavour. Put them into a food mixer with a little coconut or almond milk and whizz up until it is ice-cream texture.

Maybe a Smoothie made with a few oats, fresh fruit and seeds will go down well.

You can also offer little bowls of raisins, unsweetened dried mango or pineapple, with cashew or almond nuts, and pumpkin and sunflower seeds for them to nibble. Young children should not be given whole nuts/seeds, particularly peanuts, which are not true nuts anyway.

Children will love these special treats.

Try to make food special and appetising without resorting to crisps, sweets, fizzy drinks, or chocolate. Meat, eggs and fish are not necessary when a child is congested. **Avoid sugar, wheat and cheese** as much as possible. Milk shakes are not a good idea as **milk is mucous forming**.

Although having a cold may make a child less interested in food, it is a good idea to encourage a light healthy diet during the course of a heavy cold. It will keep their Energy up and always ensure they have plenty of liquids.

Garlic is a wonderful natural antibiotic, and antifungal. It can be put into soup and vegetable stews, or stir fries but as it has a very strong flavour don't force it on your child in a raw state except in very small quantities. It may be palatable raw with some honey and cider vinegar mixed with it, once it is well crushed. Give a small teaspoonful of this like medicine, just taking the juice.

Manuka honey, from New Zealand, is full of healing enzymes, and though expensive to buy, can be spread thinly on rice cakes as a treat when the child is poorly.

Elder, as found in hedgerows, with white flowers in the late spring, is a wonderful treatment for colds and coughs. You can try making your own Elderflower cordial, using honey as sweetener. Dilute a little of the cordial in warm water with a slice of lemon. It makes a cold clear up quicker and loosens mucous. Elder Berries can be collected in early autumn and a cordial made by steeping them in hot water, honey, ginger and cloves. The rich purple syrup makes a great cough mixture. You can find quite a few different recipes on-line.

Root Ginger, though rather an adult taste, is very cleansing to the system and stimulates the warmth of the body to overcome the bugs itself. It can be chopped up finely in soups or a slice in hot water can make an interesting drink with lemon and honey.

Vitamin C is well known as a remedy for colds/coughs. It boosts the immune system. It can be found in fresh fruit, especially oranges/ Satsuma and rosehips and also fresh vegetables not overcooked. Taking a supplement of Vit C throughout the cold winter months can help keep colds at bay. Get a good one from the local health food shop, especially for children, and ask the assistant for help on dosage.

Echinacea is becoming better known as a winter remedy to boost the immune system. It can be taken by children and is most efficacious as drops. Again check with the assistant about the best dosage for your child.

Mustard sounds like a real Granny Recipe, but can be very good at times. Put a deep bowl of hot water on the floor on a towel, add about a dessertspoon of mustard powder, and get the child to sit still with their feet in the bowl. Sit beside them and read a story. Once the skin begins to pink up, gently dry off their legs/feet and massage with nice oil and put on woolly socks. This can be a super treatment for a tired cold child who wants a bit of TLC (tender loving care!) and helps with the stuffed up head feeling as it draws the warmth down. Try it yourself if you have a cold.

An older child can have a **steam inhalation.**

If the cold becomes really heavy and sinuses are painful and blocked, steam can be used to help clear the passages.

Great care must be taken with this, and the child must be well supervised.

Boil a kettle of water and pour into a large basin. Add a chamomile tea bag, or better still a few **loose chamomile** flowers. Also Vick, eucalyptus oil or Friars Balsam can be used in small quantities for really blocked sinuses.

Settle the child down next to a table so they can lean over the hot bowl. Put a towel right over their heads, so that the steam comes up onto their face and get them to breathe deeply, let them stay under the towel for at least 5 minutes, longer if they will.

Afterwards dry their face and make sure they do not go out into a cold atmosphere for a while. They can also have a good blow with tissues, as this loosens the mucous.

The steam is very soothing and healing to the inflamed sinuses.

With a young child, setting up a steamer in the bedroom can be really helpful at night, especially if they are prone to **croup**, which is a spasm of the throat, and can obstruct breathing and be very frightening to both the parents and child. Herbal oils, such as eucalyptus or lavender can be added to ease the congestion.

If your child is unfortunate enough to get **ear problems** these can also be eased using natural methods. Firstly ensure that your child wears a good woollen hat when they go out with a cold. Cold air onto an already inflamed system will create more inflammation.

Ears and the tube between the throat and ears may get blocked with mucous and middle ear infections may occur. These are incredibly painful and a screaming child may need to be held and comforted in your bed or on your lap. Giving Kalpol for this is not unreasonable as earache is one of the worst pains.

An extremely useful treatment may be done with a large **onion.**

Cut the onion into fairly thick slices and store in the fridge. Take one large slice, wrap it well in a cotton handkerchief and place it over the painful ear. Put on a hat or head scarf to keep it in place and encourage the child to rest quietly in bed lying on the affected side, with possibly a warm hot water bottle as well placed on the ear.

The onion actually 'draws out' the inflammation and this may avoid a ruptured eardrum or glue ear developing. Glue ear is when the mucous becomes sticky and sucks in the ear drum causing hearing loss. It is treated most often by inserting grommets, small 'pegs' which break the vacuum between the outer and inner ear.

If the child is obviously ill, with a temperature, delirium or the pain is not subsiding it may be a case of needing an antibiotic, so make an appointment to see a doctor urgently, but try an onion first as it often works!

Chest complications after a cold are also fairly common. The cough, rather than being loose and tickly will become heavy with a rattle. At this stage a fever may develop.

Observing your child and allowing them to rest quietly at home may avoid further problems and they will gradually improve with a good diet, fluids and care. However if they get a fever, or the cough is much worse or they are breathless, you could try a chest poultice. The easiest is made with lemons.

Cut up a **large lemon** (organic) under warm water until the juices of both skin and pulp are running. Get a large cotton handkerchief and put into the water. Wring it out well, so it is not dripping and place right around the child's chest. Cover immediately with a layer of warm wool, and get them to rest lying down for at least 2 hours. Remove the poultice and repeat as necessary. The lemon draws out the inflammation.

This can also be done with old fashioned kaolin poultice, as bought in good chemist shops, or with curd cheese. German '**Quark'** works well for this. It is a well-known treatment in Germany.

Resorting to antibiotics is a fairly frequent scenario, but before you get some from the GP, try to establish if the infection is viral or bacterial. Antibiotics only work on bacterial infections.

Many antibiotics nowadays are becoming ineffectual as bugs are becoming 'superbugs'. Therefore giving them unnecessarily only makes this problem worse. I have read that antibiotics may become a thing of the past in a few years' time.

When you have a cold you feel rotten and so this is NOT the time to be sent to nursery or school. Many parents take the attitude 'Oh, it's ONLY a cold' and children will be sent off with streaming noses or coughs. Much better to keep the child in an even temperature for 24-48 hours until the worst symptoms have passed. Catching a cold is an indicator that the immune system is under stress and the child needs a bit more 'Mummy time'.

Our present government is pushing for all mothers to be able to work. They are supporting financially those who want to send their children to nursery.

I recently read of a Swedish research project which studied older children who had been brought up in state-run nurseries. They consistently showed more psychological problems, more addictive behaviour and more depression and violent tendencies than those who had stayed at home with the parents.

It is hard to stick out against the 'norms in society', especially when there are also financial incentives to do otherwise.

'Grannies remedies' did us well for many hundreds of years and we may well have to resort back to them again in the future, when nature is the only cure.

The very simplest and best thing you can do for your child is make sure they stay WARM when their bodies are in an inflammatory state with a cold or cough. Allow them to rest more and reduce their activity programme to a minimum. That way only does the body have a chance to rebalance and heal itself; as it surely will, given the right environment.

Fevers

The next stage on from a cough or cold is a full-blown fever. Fevers can be due to a bacterium in the blood or an acute viral infection such as influenza, or a so-called 'childhood illness' or a complication of a cold such as ear infections or bronchitis. A small child with a high fever can be a very frightening thing, as they go quickly into a state of crisis. Other symptoms are usually present to give a clue as to the nature of the illness.

The child may well want to sleep. They look very flushed and may also become delirious. Their breathing may become shallow, they may be a little blue around the lips, or they may have a febrile convulsion. This is a serious side effect of high fever in young children.

Taking the child's temperature is necessary to recognise the severity of the illness. This can be done with an oral thermometer in older children, or up the bottom, or under the arm in younger ones. The best easiest temperature gauges are those that simply go on the forehead and give an almost instant reading. These can be bought in chemist shops and are an essential part of any family's first aid kit. If you are caught out without a thermometer a good instant check can be done by putting your hand on their forehead. It will feel much hotter than usual.

If the child has a fever of 1-2 degrees centigrade (no higher than 39C) then there is no need to panic. Make sure the child is dressed in warm cotton/wool clothing and try to get them settled somewhere where they can lie quietly. This could be a sofa in the lounge where you are sitting quietly, a little bed in the dining room on an inflatable mattress where they can see you cooking or washing dishes, or it may be their own beds, providing they are given a little bell to call you, or you pop in and out frequently. Children do not like to be left alone when ill, and should also not be left in case the fever rises sharply. Just sitting and cuddling them for hours can be the most soothing beneficial thing for them. Ensure the house is kept a warm even temperature and that you have someone else to do the school pickups, shopping or whatever needs doing out and about. Your prime task is to create a 'Huelle' (a German word meaning a wrapped up cosy space), within which your child can relax and feel totally nurtured and safe.

Time heals and your child will be busy healing whatever the problem, given the right environment.

Ensure they take enough liquids, as a fevered body quickly gets very dehydrated, and offer only fruit puree or small pieces of fruit for the first 24 hours. The digestion probably needs a rest too. Giving them some ice to suck on can be soothing too, but avoid cold ice creams at first. As the temperature goes down you can start a light diet as offered for a cold, with no sugar, wheat or dairy, or additives whatsoever.

If the fever is rising above 39-40c and the child is beginning to look ill, getting a fan to cool them down can help. Also gently sponging them down with a sponge dipped in lemon water (as made for cold compresses above) will bring down a fever. Another good way is to bring the temperature down to the feet by wrapping the calves up in a cloth containing either quark or squeezed out lemon clothes. The child must have these on for several hours and they can be changed regularly. Not all children will have a fit if the temperature rises. My youngest son had a temperature of 43c once with no ill effect!

However use your powers of observation and instincts to know whether the process is sustainable or not. Calling the doctor might set your mind at rest or might involve an antibiotic injection or even admission to hospital

Some things to look out for, at which you will need to call medical help

- A febrile convulsion or fit
- Severe headache
- Stiff neck or sensitivity to light,
- Extreme dehydration from vomiting/diarrhoea.
- Any unusual rashes which are not explained as measles, rubella, chickenpox.

Check out the symptoms of the childhood illnesses if you have decided not to inoculate and the child may have been in contact with them, so you know just what you are dealing with. Measles must be carefully nursed as the secondary meningitis infections; ear or eye problems may cause difficulties if you do not keep the child quietly resting. Most problems that one hears about are due to poor nursing and pushing the child back to school too quickly.

New varieties of childhood illnesses are appearing as a result of mass inoculation, which means that symptoms may not follow a very typical pattern. In this scenario your doctor can advise as he knows what is going around, and the illness picture which is presenting.

Young children will often spike a temperature if they are **teething.** This needs rather different treatment, as the work the child is doing changing/cutting their teeth is a fundamental development, which needs space, time and understanding. Some children sail through this, others become quite ill and restless. Giving **homeopathic Chamomile drops in a little water** will act as a soothing help for this process.

Using Homeopathic remedies can be incredibly efficacious when a child is ill. Knowing what to give when and how each remedy is suited to a particular child can be confusing initially. If you become interested in this deep subject it is worth taking your child to a qualified homeopath and asking them which remedies would suit them for a fever. There may be other developmental issues which can be really helped by giving these little sugar pills or drops. They have no side effects and can be surprisingly potent.

A common one used for fever, when the child's face is flushed and the eyes look glazed is **Belladonna,** but this will not be the remedy of choice for all children.

Whatever else happens, remaining calm with a sick child is of the utmost importance. Put your life on hold for however long it takes and try not to have selfish restless thoughts about what you are missing of REAL life! Life is real enough for you in the sick room and it is the very best most important thing you can do for your child. It teaches you patience by the bucket load!

I remember my mother nursing me and my sister through first mumps and then measles. We had them in succession and she was stuck at home for 12 weeks! Friends came to visit and even came to babysit on occasion which we loved, but she never ditched out on us, or sent us back to school too soon! It must have been a real life lesson. Thank you, Mum.

Accidents and injuries

Before I start on the practicalities I am going to say a strange thing; "Nothing happens by accident!"

By this I mean that the child will become involved in whatever trauma that befalls him/her and on a deeply subconscious level will know why this is happening to them. They may need the 'stop' that an accident brings and any lessons they learn from going through this experience will be valuable to them on a developmental level.

They may be craving more love and attention; they may have become over-restless and inattentive to what their bodies are doing. Or there may be a deeper level on which this occurs which we cannot even start to judge or understand. These may seem callous and strange words indeed, but ponder them and glimpses of understanding may start to appear. I do not believe in an angry God who punishes, but that everything in the world has a natural pattern of Energy flow.

Some children are very accident prone and always breaking bones and going off to E and A, to the extent that some parents have even been accused of neglect by the hospital staff.

I am not intimating this at all! Having had one son who was often in casualty, it 'just happened'; but WHY?

The first reaction of a parent in an accident is usually huge shock and fear. Try if possible to learn to trust a process and remain calm in the face of the pain of your loved ones. That way you can give more love and support. What is your biggest fear? Always ask that question and face it. Many conflicting emotions may be present too. Guilt, anger, blame, shock, disbelief, but the greatest one is fear.

Make sure you know what to do in any given situation. The role of the parent often involves being a first-aider and practical skills are sometimes important. Get a good book and study it or go on a paediatric first aid course.

In your first aid box you should have not only the normal selection of sterile dressings and plasters, but a bottle of **Bach's 'Rescue Remedy'**; herbal drops in brandy which you put on your tongue every few minutes if necessary and can also give to your child. It can also be put on the temples or wrists. This is calming and helps you feel more in control.

Arnica D6 is a well-known homeopathic home treatment for shocks, bruising and tumbles. The little white pills can be bought in most good pharmacies and should be sucked under the tongue until dissolved. You can give these immediately and then continue for a few days after the accident until the child is more steady and less traumatised, taking it 3-4 times a day. It also comes as a tincture, which can be used diluted in boiled water as a compress for bruises and sprains, or as a cream to be put on bumps and bruises. **Never** put arnica on an open wound or graze, or use it when the skin is broken.

If the child has a dirty graze or cut, clean it very well first under running water or bathe it gently in cool boiled water that has some **Calendula lotion** added. This is made from marigolds and is a wonderful natural antiseptic. **Diluted Witch-hazel** is also good. It is important to remove all the grit and dirt before putting on a dry sterile dressing. Calendula cream is also available, or use a mild antiseptic cream without too many additives.

Keeping a frozen pad in the freezer to put onto sprains and bruises is a useful thing. Frozen peas are almost as good!

Sometimes it is hard to know if a wound needs stitches. As a rule of thumb try to bring together the edges of a wound as tightly as you can using 'steristrip' plasters. If you are unsure, or the wound is jagged or in an awkward place, or near eyes or mouth, take the child to be sutured professionally. Scaring will develop from a badly healed wound, which they will not thank you for in the future.

Burns, if mild, should be treated by running under cold water immediately. I keep an Aloe Vera plant on my kitchen window sill and the juice from a leaf broken off can be smeared directly onto a burn or scald and works really well. It can also be put onto burned tongues after hot liquid! Any large or severe burns need professional care.

If **glass** is involved in an accident never try to remove it from the limb but take the child straight to hospital. Taking the glass out might cause serious blood loss.

If you think the child has **broken a limb** try to keep it as still as possible strapped to their body. You can improvise a sling or splint with a scarf or tea towel.

Shock, when the blood pressure drops and the child is white and semiconscious from blood loss or trauma is serious; always call emergency help if the child has lost a lot of blood or seems to have an internal injury.

If the child has a **head bump** observe them carefully for several hours afterwards and don't let them go to sleep in case there has been some internal damage. Uneven pupil size or drowsiness needs immediate medical attention.

It is often difficult to assess if you need to take your child to hospital. Children get bumps and bruises as a normal part of growing up, but a child's cry will often indicate how severe their damage is. Sometimes there is a horrible silence after a fall and then you know that immediate action is needed. If the child is very upset emotionally don't over-fuss but give them diversion or calm cuddles and it will soon pass. You know your child best and instinct is often the best guide.

If you think the child has broken something or may need surgery of some kind or an anaesthetic, don't let them eat or drink anything until you are sure. Delayed treatment because the child has eaten within 4 hours can be crucial in the healing process.

Remember that any trauma will shock the child on a deep level. This means that they will need rest, quiet and your healing presence to help them recover. This may take a few days. Sometimes a child will even get a temperature after an accident, as part of the shock to their system. A light diet and a few treats will help to make them feel special and loved and recover quicker.

Your own Energy as a parent is transferred to them when you give love, cuddles and comfort. You are acting as a **Healer** to your child and this action cannot be underestimated.

Giving Love unconditionally at such times is the greatest gift to your children. Fear is the opposite of love and feeling fear prevents you from giving your full love, so work on overcoming your fears to help your child when they experience trauma of any kind.

Tummy upsets

These are very common in young children and are usually caused by a 'bug' or virus which the child has come into contact with. Washing hands before eating and after using the toilet is an important lesson to teach a child from an early age and will minimise the risk of catching an infection. Tummy upsets may occasionally be caused by food poisoning and the suspect meal needs to be traced if possible.

Allergic reactions to certain foods can also induce tummy upsets, which can be quite extreme. Keep a note of any repeated episodes, and ask your doctor/health visitor if you are concerned.

The strengthening of the immune system through good general care and diet will help also in fighting off any bugs which are going the rounds at nursery or school, or mean that the infection will pass quickly through the system and leave the child little affected by it.

Conversely a weak child may become very ill quite quickly if they lose vital body fluids through vomiting or diarrhoea and this may then become a medical emergency and admission to hospital for rehydration may be needed.

A young baby can quickly lose fluids, and this is obvious by lassitude and the fontanel (soft spot) caving inwards. In this case call a doctor.

Normally the child vomits as the body's natural mechanism to clear the system of toxic waste; as is also diarrhoea, so it can be seen as a cleansing process. The child needs to be supported in this in the same way as with any illness, with quiet rest and sips of water. It is best to **rest the digestion** completely to begin with and only give a rice cake (with no butter) of the child says they are hungry.

How long should you starve them? For 24 hours after an acute attack of sickness or diarrhoea only give water or herbal tea, (chamomile is especially soothing and should be made weak with no sweetening) and then gradually introduce a light non-fatty diet, like some vegetable soup or fruit puree, or some porridge.

If the child is sick again, reduce the amount of food given and wait and watch! If a tummy bug lasts for more than 2-3 days and there seems to be no sign of improvement you should contact medical advice, as a child may become dehydrated. Giving sachets of rehydration powder, containing vital electrolytes can sometimes be a good idea if they are very sick and weak, but don't ignore the symptoms if they go on longer than a couple of days.

The symptoms of **appendicitis** are worth being aware of. Tummy ache which can be severe is usually felt across the middle of the abdomen, around the umbilicus. It may also cause sickness. If the child complains often of tummy ache of this kind or has a temperature with severe tummy ache, don't ignore it. Burst appendix is not uncommon and may be life threatening.

Tummy ache can also be a sign of **emotional tension**. Some children are more prone to it than others. Having wind pockets or just sore feelings in the abdomen may indicate nervous tension and a digestive weakness. Helping the child to be calm at mealtimes, with no toys, distractions, TV or rows and to sit down throughout the meal may help a nervy child to digest better. Massaging the abdomen gently can be very soothing in this scenario; the child may like to lie down on their front with a pillow under their tummy.

Recurring tummy aches can also be an attention seeking ploy, so look at things like relationship issues in the family, school bullying, or general unhappiness for some reason. A sympathetic chat at bedtime can often sort out problems of this kind and make the child feel more supported.

In normal good health we are not aware of the digestive tract and its workings. Only of there is inflammation or disease do we become aware of what is going on in this highly complex and important part of our bodies. The subconscious metabolism then becomes conscious; hence if there are emotional, nervous issues these can also be felt in the abdominal area.

In this section I have tried to cover all the common problems which may occur day by day when one has a young family. There are detailed and excellent books available on first aid and childhood illnesses, and having a small reference library will help you to diagnose and treat these common problems yourself with more confidence. The GPs and health visitors are there as back-up for you if you are concerned or the child is not recovering spontaneously. Have trust that young bodies **do heal** spontaneously and well, given the right calm environment and diet. Your task as a parent is to support that natural process with intuition, calmness and love.

Rhythm and warmth

As we discussed in Part 1 the child's Energy is closely associated with MOVEMENT and LIFE. The **pulse**, which we take so for granted, is the sign that the heart is alive, and it maintains a steady and unwavering tempo throughout our entire lives. Only when the heartbeat stops are we dead! The heart muscle is the strongest in the body and starts to beat even before the heart as an organ is fully formed in the embryo. This is a strange miracle worth pondering. The beat is there before the organ; in fact the organ is formed BY the beat!

Another miracle of life is the sustaining of **warmth.** The warmth of mammals has developed gradually over time. Dinosaurs, fish and birds have a very different kind of heat mechanism. The blood sustains and nourishes every cell in our warm bodies, and pulses with life throughout every cell, renewing and sustaining our processes.

Without warmth we quickly die. If we get too hot we can also die. We take these things for granted, but it is worth thinking about if you are a parent responsible for maintaining the warmth of a baby or young child, or even a teenager!

The surface skin area of humans is covered with sweat glands and fine hairs, which help to even out changes in temperature, but in our fickle climate we also have to wear varying amounts of clothes and have heating in our houses. If we ignore this need we can soon become ill.

The head has a large surface area and as much as an **eighth of your body heat can be lost** rapidly through your head. If a child gets cold regularly they also have to utilise their own Energy to maintain body heat; Energy which should be going towards growth and development in a young child.

From this perspective one can begin to understand how some of the British habits of the last century of dressing children in shorts and ankle socks throughout cold winters may have contributed to the large numbers of elderly people now who have got arthritic knees and hips in this country! The Energy which should have been used to develop strong limbs went into keeping them warm, thus weakening the child as they grew older.

How often does one see babies with bare heads nowadays out in the cold wind? Yes, they survive but at what hidden costs? How often can you hear a young child crying from cold on a windy day down by the sea? Keeping our children warm is rather like keeping a precious plant in the green-house. If you put it out in a cold draught too early in spring it will curl up and die, but if you keep it indoors on a hot day it will become lanky and yellow and eventually die also. Our children are no different. We need the right balance of warmth and wrapping to keep them healthy. Overdressing will not allow them to move and use their limbs, but underdressing, which is the bigger problem, weakens their Energy and can cause illness and frailty later.

Clothes made of natural fibres which breathe and allow the child to sweat naturally with layers of cotton and wool is best. If artificial dressings are put into the clothes to 'keep them fresh' this also may affect the ability of the skin to act as a natural organ of excretion, which it is. Nylon, acrylic and other artificial fabrics are best avoided altogether.

Rhythm is an interesting topic as it is largely hidden in our bodies, but every process has its own rhythm. There are rhythms of the liver and gall bladder, the hormones, the sleep mechanisms and many other bodily systems. Everything gyrates together in harmony rather like a huge 'Dance of Energy'. From a parents' perspective it is therefore helpful for your growing child to sustain and maintain these natural rhythms.

Bedtime should be at the same time each night, preferably early for young children, as sleep is vital, mealtimes should be regular, the pattern of the week can also be developed with special things on special days, so the child comes to recognise the 7 day rhythm which is also not just incidental.

The seasonal rhythms can be celebrated also. These are ancient points in the year when certain rituals were done, dating back to the Druids and even earlier, when people knew intuitively about the cycles of the sun, moon and stars. Our modern Christian festivals are loosely connected to the cycles of the seasons. In Mediaeval times the rent was collected on quarter days. The Celtic festivals recognise these dates also, with midsummer, midwinter, spring and autumn equinox. Harvest, All Souls, or Halloween and May Day are all markers of these yearly cycles.

Doing fun and creative rituals, appropriate to each age group, on these festivals can help the child to connect more strongly to the natural seasonal changes. Their awareness of the earth and its seasons helps to strengthen the body's rhythms also.

A healthy child is one who connects in a natural way with its environment and its cultural inheritance. It absorbs this unconsciously in the early years from its parents and wider family. If this is disrupted or not recognised the child can feel unsettled and not have a deep connectedness or sense of 'home' to the place on earth where it is brought up. In later life this can show as restlessness, many moves and a weakening of the natural rhythms of the bodily functions, such as sleep, which may then cause illnesses to develop.

Rhythm in the widest meaning can also be found in music and beat. Children who have an early environment where music is heard and practised develop their sense of natural rhythm. Dance is another way to do this. Research has shown that children who play an instrument and sing have a higher IQ and find concentration easier. The brain develops more fully when natural rhythms and tones are introduced early on.

Sleep disturbances

I would particularly like to mention here the ever increasing problem of **sleep** in our modern children. Having initially been invited to take part in the TV programme 'Bedtime Live' recently, but then declined, I watched with horror some of the scenarios which were being tackled by the 'experts'.

A child, who has natural 'organic' rhythms (i.e. who during the day eats **good food** regularly, plays in a **calm environment,** has plenty of **fresh air and exercise** in the right amounts, who is kept the **right temperature** and dressed well, who has plenty of contact with their parents in a **relaxed happy loving** space and who has had a normal relaxed **birth** with no complications, and has been **breastfed** well,) will normally go to bed happily and sleep for up to 12 hours a night!

Problems with sleep often start very early on, and then may need professional help to sort them out later. If a baby is carried downstairs and stimulated in the early weeks every time it cries, its night/day rhythms will not get well established. Because food is a new experience to a baby's body, the timing, quantity and quality of feeds helps to establish these natural rhythms. Therefore complete demand feeding as has become popular is perhaps not helping our children to sleep. Chemical cow's milk formulas may also have a bearing on sleep quality as it is digested differently, and car rides and TV watching must also overstimulate the child's nerve-sense system.

Rigidity in a parent is not good, and anxiety is even worse! Many children will settle happily with a grandparent or nanny but will play up over-anxious parents. This is not just a statement from my personal experience but also the tales of many of my older female friends which leads me to write this! Fashions in childrearing go in cycles, and we seem to have experimented a lot with our children in the last 20-30 years.

It is helpful to have a **bedtime routine** to enable the child to wind down after a busy day. Many children cannot sleep because they are overtired and overstimulated.

The routine could include a warm bath, with some lavender bath oil to relax them, and some water play. Mum or Dad must always be there calmly enjoying this time with their children. Rushing off to cook a meal, answering the phone or whatever disrupts the child.

The child's evening meal, with a parent eating too, must be taken early with just a warm drink at bedtime, as the digestion needs time to settle before sleep. Waiting up for Dad to come back from work and then bouncing around in play can disrupt the settling.

Getting into bed, without any TV or radio in the room, with a soft cover and some special cuddly toy, but not too many bright garish stimulating pictures on the walls or covers, one can then tell a story, simple and repetitive for young children, imaginative, while you cuddle them gently or perhaps a book read each night for an older child; then a brief chat about the day, some sharing time or perhaps stroking the child's head gently, until they are ready to let you go downstairs.

A song and a candle to create a quiet atmosphere can also be calming. The light goes out and the door is shut, from an early age, with no arguments! Minimal fuss or anxiety or going in and out after settling will give the child security and a strong message that they don't play up! If you are sure in yourself that the child will sleep it invariably will.

Occasionally a baby may have had a traumatic birth, as in a caesarean or forceps and then a cranial-sacral osteopathic treatment may be helpful. This is a very gentle and non-invasive treatment that encourages the cerebrospinal fluids to move more harmoniously. This happens at a normal birth, but may become disrupted if there are birth delays or no natural passage through the birth canal. It can have a dramatic effect on settling the baby into a calmer routine.

Another time that sleep may become disrupted is if the child has an unnatural separation from the parents through a hospital admission of the mother or child. In this case quiet perseverance using gradual separation techniques can help an anxious child to settle again. Patience and love will be needed, and a set pattern which never changes.

If you want your child to sleep in your bed, you will allow it too, but don't expect it to suddenly disappear again! Set the rules you want from the outset. Children just like animals can be trained providing you stay calm and focused. Talk about problems with your health visitor and make sure you have a united front with your husband/wife.

I had a son who did not want to stay in his cot at the age of 14 months. It took 3 nights (and my husband being persuaded by both the GP and health visitor) to get him not to stand up and scream, but after that he slept perfectly, and never played up again.

Finding your boundaries with a small child is a two-way process and involves much patience, humour, insight and love. The path of parenting is a path of personal development.

Emotional problems

Our society reflects very much what is going on in each and every home throughout the country. Bringing up healthy emotionally balanced children is the basis for the next generation and how they create a future community, both in terms of work, ethics and morals, and also as future parents themselves. As parents we are constantly learning from our children if we can remain alert and open to what they innately bring. We do have to help and guide them however.

Any routine and house rules are part of the relationship you create with your child, which starts early on, even in utero. How much do you demand and how much do they get their own way? There seem to be two extremes and society tends to swing like a pendulum between these two.

If a child is over regimented and not allowed to express its uniqueness and grow into its own personality, it will be suppressed and unable to express its natural gifts. It may suffer from constipation or nervous stress in later life, or be unable to initiate things and feel low self-esteem or depression as an adult. Controlling parents often breed controlling children, unless the individual realises this and compensates for its upbringing.

A child who does not have any consistency or rules will suffer as well. Many children in our current society are in this situation, offspring off the '60's kids'. Parents do their children no favours with a totally 'laise faire' attitude, as boundaries give children a sense of security. These children may grow up trying drugs or over-binging on alcohol, and may find it hard to hold down a regular job in later life, or take responsibility for parenting themselves.

One of the keys to nurturing a young child is to help them to feel a **sense of wonder** and **devotion** to all things natural and beautiful. The world is a beautiful place with huge diversity of creatures and plants which we have a responsibility to care for. If we drop litter, squash flies, kick the dog, disregard and neglect our patch of garden, use foul language and get angry easily we are giving strong messages to our children. We are **literally teaching them aggression and lack of love.**

It is not just a 'social class' phenomenon, how we talk to and treat our children. Every human being has it in them to be loving, gentle, kind and patient. Nowadays one of the greatest negative influences on our young children is the constant bombardment of ugly and aggressive images from the television. Even cartoons like Tom and Jerry (fun as they may seem to an adult) are aggressive and distorted. The animals are not true animals, but are distortions of human beings. If a young child, who acts as a complete **sponge** to everything around them, watches television, not only is their concentration span diminished as they watch constantly flashing changing images, but they are taking in on a deep level the distorted image of the human being. Huge eyes, little legs, enormous mouths, angular 'disabled' bodies. Watch some children's programmes and you will see it for yourself!

For parents TV is a wonderful 'babysitter'. A child will sit quietly for hours not disturbing you while you chat to a friend on the phone or make a meal, or even work at the computer! Instead of talking and relating to you, their parent, and learning about the skills of life and attitudes and love, our children are put into a semi-conscious state (the same part of the brain is used for watching TV as when we are unconscious) and given the equivalent of pornography to watch! These may sound strong words, but I have seen time and time again how children react after they have watched some television. They are restless, maybe flushed, cannot concentrate and start acting out the aggressive behaviour they have been watching.

Multiply this by hundreds of hours over the years and we are breeding a generation of brainwashed children who have short concentration spans, learned aggressive behaviour, lack of communication skills; and a sense that the world of 'illusion', is in fact reality.

Electronic games and computer education is having a similar effect on our children. They are becoming more and more brain orientated, as is the whole of our society, and their bodies and imaginations, and emotional responses are becoming stultified. It is not only in homes that we find this, but more and more teaching is now done on computers, and children are expected to download 'facts' from the endless resources now available to regurgitate them as learning. How little this has to do with 'real life', the cycles of nature, the interaction of human beings and the development of compassion, empathy and love.

What are we doing it for? Simply to respond to peer group pressure? Or to keep them quiet? Or to 'educate' them? If you are experiencing ANY disturbance or problems with your children's behaviour or sleep, the very first thing to try is to 'break' the TV! Make it disappear (maybe up to your bedroom, into a cupboard, if **you** are still addicted!) Keep TV, electronic games and computers absolutely out of their lives and you will be amazed at the gradual changes that occur; in behaviour, communication, sleep patterns and physical health and robustness!

Sure, you as the guiding adult or teacher will have to supply other games and pastimes. Perhaps a large sandpit for a young child in the garden, some pots of paints, baking times in the kitchen, hide and seek, cutting and sticking, a climbing frame and swing, regular walks, a pet to learn to care for, some beautiful story books (not a repetition of the distortion from the TV characters!) or some building materials. Children between 3 and 7 love to build houses and camps, play families, and play with dolls. The child learns by acting out what it sees around it. They COPY everything and then practise it. That is their work! Constructing wooden towers at an early age can help them develop balance and coordination.

It is not necessary to do endless puzzles and 'educational' games to develop life skills. Climbing trees, learning to play an instrument, drawing with big colourful crayons, can allow the child to breathe out and develop their bodies more fully throughout childhood, which is the vital time for this. Computers and facts can be easily acquired when needed at a later stage.

If you sit all day at a computer the child will want to do likewise; if you bake something interesting, the child will want to copy you. If you sew and knit, the child will soon want to learn. If you make lots of tea and chat to your friends, the child will play this out in their Wendy house. This may seem obvious, but YOU are the measure of their world to begin with. They are busy from morning till night learning how to be like you.

That is the greatest compliment you will get as a parent, and you will soon perceive how they have 'absorbed' you. Do they drop litter or pick it up, do they say thank you and please, do they sit quietly at the table and eat their food, do they take an interest in visitors and smile and greet them with confidence, do they keep their rooms looking nice, do they go to sleep easily at night, do they show an interest in nature and animals or plants? All these attributes are learned by COPYING.

You cannot expect your child to be polite if you shout at them to reprimand them, or even slap them. You cannot want them to be concentrated and peaceful if you are restless and easily bored; you cannot tell them off for quarrelling with their brothers or sisters if you quarrel with your partner!

Just as they are learning from you, so too you are learning from them. If you hit a big problem, and there can be many as the years go on, first look at what is going on in YOU, and see if you can change that first. If you are anxious or depressed find out why. What is your fear? Are you unsupported, lacking self-love, angry, or low in self-esteem?

No-one is perfect and neither are your children. The personality of your child, their unique gifts and qualities and also their problems are obvious to you if you really observe them from a very early age.

As a parent you can adjust your attitudes and parameters to suit each child. Listen to what they are telling you, even in their first cries, and demands. That is not about giving in to their every demand, but understanding their pain of being human too. You can feel in empathy their frustration and fear, you can try to overcome that same frustration and fear in yourself.

This may all sound very idealistic, but it is the ground on which you build your child's future emotional health. Listening to advice from others can be very confusing as each person carries their own fears, built in from childhood, and the best way to help your child in their problems is to look inside yourself and use your **intuition** to understand what is happening.

Sometimes sharing your own growth with a close friend or counsellor may be helpful. At each stage of childhood and parenting the child can show us another aspect of ourselves.

Some people love caring for babies. They are naturally maternal/paternal and enjoy the demands and cuddles needed. The baby is totally helpless and innocent.

Others will find this stage challenging and boring and long for the baby to become a little person with whom they can talk and play. Watching them develop their first words and faltering steps, likes and dislikes can be fascinating.

Other people prefer a school age child who is exploring the world out there, and comes back from school with new knowledge. They enjoy helping to teach and guide their children.

Others find the challenges of teenagers stimulating and interesting, as the young person flexes their emotional muscles ready to 'leave the nest', and more and more tries to realise their ideals in a concrete way. Many of our teenagers are very angry and disillusioned at the adults they see around them.

Whatever stage you enjoy and whichever bits of parenting you personally find challenging, sharing your journey with others, your partner, teachers, friends and family, can be a support and help.

Having had the experience of being a single parent of three children myself, I cannot say too strongly how support is helpful and necessary. We were not intended to live in isolation, as nuclear families. If you observe all indigenous peoples (and also primates in the wild) you can see how family/community support is part of growing up healthily. Grandparents (and aunts and uncles) are important to enable children to have a sense of family history and continuum, and Grannies too can develop a unique relationship with their grandchildren. Other friends with children of similar ages can provide extra 'siblings', particularly if you have an only child. Doing swaps during the holidays and weekends can bring new dimensions into your family life and also give you a few hours to yourself when needed.

The assumption that parents have the greatest educational input in their children's emotional wellbeing is greatly challenged nowadays by societies' and the governments' pressure for parents to work outside the home. Homecare and childcare is totally **undervalued by our current society,** reflected in the minimal wages that nannies and housekeepers are offered. It is seen as much more important to sit at an office desk all day staring at a computer screen.

So our children are neglected and brought up haphazardly in nurseries and by child-minders, who sometimes (as experts) do a better job than the real parents. Why do we have children? Is it just a status symbol? With the rapid over population of the planet we have to seriously ask whether we are worthy of becoming real parents! The continuation of the human species relies on good parenting and also good education, whatever we take that word to mean.

With a risk of alienating you, or sending you on an unhealthy 'guilt trip', by what I am saying, I would like to point out that we have a very grave problem in our present age. Children are **emotionally deprived** throughout all of society and differing income brackets, because we do not give enough importance to giving our children **our time** and parenting skills on all levels. Earning money has become a greater priority. Only when this fact changes will we start to build a healthy society for the future of our planet.

One aspect which needs to be mentioned is the early sexuality which children are experiencing. There are several factors which may be influencing this. Children experience early stimulation with our modern environment. They are encouraged to use their nerve/sense systems more than in previous times. They are forced to sit up earlier, have long car and air journeys and have less sleep. Their diet may well influence this too, with meat containing growth hormones being fed to the animals.

Toys show sexually developed figures (such as Barbie dolls) and TV is constantly showing precocious tinies acting up (as in Hanna Montana). Children's clothes are now like baby adults ones, children wear makeup and bras much earlier, and generally children come into puberty earlier and earlier.

Children are literally being ROBBED of their childhood, a time of dreamy imagination, of play and learning about natural laws and social interaction. These lessons are being missed out on, as we rush our children headlong into an adult world of ambitions, material needs, technical and academic achievements and money making.

It may be no surprise to hear that degenerative illnesses, Alzheimer's disease and dementia are becoming ever more common at earlier ages. We do not have the oportunity to **build up** our physical bodies as children sufficiently and we are therefore weakened and this shows itself in later life as illness and early aging.

Future generations may well suffer greatly because of what we are doing **now** to our children. Despite all scientific predictions, the average lifespan may in fact start to shorten in the future, despite all the innovations of modern medicine.

Conclusion

Throughout the writing of this book I have tried to help young parents to think about **what** they are doing, rather than telling you HOW to do it!

Some of the ideas which I have written here may seem old fashioned and out of touch with reality. However I believe that our modern society has really become out of touch with reality and thus we have become a very sick society. Only by returning to basics can we start to address some of these huge problems.

With all our knowledge, medical skills, good food and hygiene are we in fact a healthier society? I believe NOT! We have in the West rising numbers of people with gross obesity, heart disease, and different cancers. More unusual illnesses like Chronic Fatigue and Fibromyalgia are on the increase. We are now facing a time where hospitals are infected with untreatable superbugs, we are threatened constantly by new pandemics, and in other parts of the world there is even graver starvation and lack of water and healthy food. The population explosion has not helped this either.

And yet we have the answers to many of these problems. We need to search again for a healthy relationship with the planet earth. We need to SIMPLIFY our lives to a point where we can grow food locally again for our needs, so that we can live by the natural seasons and enjoy the Energy of the patch of earth where we live.

Because the earth has become so sick, it may be some time and there may be much suffering before these lessons are learnt. There may be more sickness and starvation, even in the West. This may be a frightening prospect, but as parents we are establishing the next generation, and as grandparents the next after that. Life hopefully will continue for many generations to come.

But we will have to wake up to what is happening globally and each and every person will need to act in order for the tide to turn. We need to lobby MP's about agricultural policies, vote with our feet not to accept GMO in our food, only buy good sustainable local food, teach our children about nutrition and a healthy respect and devotion for nature, ensure that we all have a small patch of land to keep growing healthy composted vegetables; these actions will create change at 'ground level'!

Driving constantly around in cars, buying our food in superstores, disposing of the piles of rubbish from this shopping into land-fill, eating large amounts of meat, condoning the use of agrochemicals or artificially manufactured foods will not heal the planet or ensure our children will not starve.

All of nature is our constant responsibility. It is the ONLY thing which matters in our survival. It is not about gross manufacturing output or what is happening in the stock exchange. These are only illusions!

All money is an illusion! It is simply an exchange of Energy. If we did not have it we would be forced back to basics of exchange of skills at local level.

Each of us has gifts and talents which we can use. Enabling our children to find these in a healthy environment will enable them to continue learning about how we can change what we have created into a healthier more sustainable planet.

As parents we can teach by example. We can truly believe that there is a way forward, without wars, starvation, climate changes and suffering.

We can practice simple ecological living!

www.ingramcontent.com/pod-product-compliance
Lightning Source LLC
Chambersburg PA
CBHW080609290526
45790CB00007B/2696